cooking for diabetics

cooking for
diabetics

OVER 50 NUTRITIOUS HIGH FIBRE, LOW
FAT, LOW-SUGAR RECIPES FOR DIABETICS

MICHELLE
BERRIEDALE-JOHNSON

SELECT
EDITIONS

Select Editions imprint specially produced for Selectabook Limited

© Anness Publishing Limited 1998, 2001

Produced by Anness Publishing Limited
Hermes House
88–89 Blackfriars Road
London SE1 8HA

A CIP catalogue record for this book is available from the British Library.

Publisher: Joanna Lorenz
Senior Cookery Editor: Linda Fraser
Indexer: Pat Coward
Nutritional Analysis: Helen Daniels
Designer: Ian Sandom
Photography: James Duncan
Food for Photography: Nicola Fowler
Styling: Rosie Hopper
Cover Design: DW Design

Previously published as Healthy Eating Library: The Diabetic Cookbook

1 3 5 7 9 10 8 6 4 2

NOTES

For all recipes, quantities are given in both metric and imperial measures
and, where appropiate, measures are also given in standard cups and
spoons. Follow one set, but not a mixture, becausethey are not
interchangeable.

Standard spoon and cup measures are level.
1 tsp = 5ml, 1 tbsp = 15ml, 1 cup = 250ml/8fl oz

Australian standard tablespoons are 20ml. Australian readers should
use 3 tsp in place of 1 tbsp for measuring small quantities of gelatine,
cornflour, salt, etc.

Size 3 (medium) eggs are used unless otherwise stated.

CONTENTS

INTRODUCTION

By the time you pick up this book you (or a friend, child or parent) may already have been diagnosed as diabetic, so you may have a pretty good idea of what being diabetic is and what it involves. However, since understanding a situation is often the key to coping with it, it may be worth reviewing what you actually know.

Don't be intimidated by the wealth of rather technical information in the next few pages. The principles of dealing with diabetes are really very simple and, once you have got the hang of them, quite easy to cope with.

Most diabetics, especially those recently diagnosed, live very healthy and normal lives – some go on to excel in sports, which many non-diabetics could not dream of. So, take heart – and read on.

WHAT IS DIABETES?

The name, *diabetes mellitus*, comes from two Greek words (*diabetes* – a siphon; *mellitus* – honey, because the urine of a diabetic tastes sweet) and describes a condition in which the sugar (or glucose) circulating in the blood cannot be absorbed properly. This results in abnormally high blood glucose levels, which can cause both short- and long-term problems.

To explain in a bit more detail: Glucose (a form of sugar) is the body's main fuel – it provides us with our energy. We absorb glucose from starchy and sugary carbohydrate foods, such as potatoes, rice and beans, breads, biscuits, cakes, sugar and sweets. As we chew, enzymes in saliva start breaking down these foods, a process that is continued by the acids in the stomach. As the food progresses on into the gut, digestive juices from the pancreas and gall bladder get to work, and by the time the food reaches the bowel it has been broken down into simple particles (including glucose), which are absorbed through the bowel wall into the bloodstream. The glucose in the bloodstream moves on through the liver where much of it is stored for future use, and into body cells where it is either burned up to provide energy or stored for future use.

However, the glucose in the blood cannot enter the cells in the liver or any other part of the body unless a chemical (insulin) effectively "opens the door" into those cells. Insulin is a hormone that is manufactured in the pancreas (the glandular organ that lies behind the stomach but in front of the backbone) and stored there until rising glucose levels in the bloodstream set off a chemical reaction, which releases the insulin. Once in the bloodstream, the insulin links into the body's cells through what are called insulin receptors (a procedure which is rather like two space ships docking). This linkage precipitates chemical changes in the cell walls, which allow the glucose through into the cell where it can be converted into energy.

In a non-diabetic this monitoring and replenishment process happens automatically so that the body's cells are continually fed with sufficient glucose for their energy needs, while excess glucose is stored in the cells. In a diabetic the system fails either because the pancreas does not produce any insulin at all (Insulin Dependent Diabetes Mellitus or IDDM) or because the pancreas' supply of insulin is reduced, the supply of insulin receptors is reduced or neither functions very efficiently (Non Insulin Dependent Diabetes or NIDDM).

Despite years of research no one has discovered why it is that the pancreas should (as in the onset of IDDM) suddenly cease to produce insulin, although it would appear that some people can have a genetic predisposition to diabetes. For susceptible individuals, a viral disease can act on the immune system to make it turn upon the "beta" cells in the pancreas, which manufacture the insulin, and destroy them. In NIDDM there seems to be not only a genetic but a radical predis-

Above: Children and young adults are more likely to be insulin dependent diabetics than non insulin dependent diabetics.

position: NIDDM is four times more common in Asian communities than in the rest of the population of Britain, for example. However, with NIDDM, which occurs mainly in older and frequently overweight people (IDDM usually occurs in thin children and people under 30), there does appear to be a link with obesity. Other possible contributory causes to NIDDM in later years could be pancreatic damage through surgery or alcohol abuse; glucose intolerance during pregnancy, which may disappear after the baby is born but leaves a predisposition to diabetes during later pregnancies or in later life; long-term use of some steroids, which raise the amount of glucose in the blood; and overactivity of the thyroid.

DIAGNOSIS AND SYMPTOMS

Diagnosis of insulin dependent diabetes is normally fairly straightforward as the symptoms, although varied, are pretty obvious and can even be quite dramatic. Non insulin dependent diabetes is another matter, since the fall in insulin production may occur over a number of years and the symptoms may be quite slight. Some people with NIDDM have no symptoms at all.

DIAGNOSIS

If you go to a doctor complaining of any of these symptoms (right), he or she will normally check for diabetes.

The first test might be for excess glucose in the urine although, since the glucose levels in the urine tend to fluctuate (and some people have a low threshold so register as having above the normal level without actually being diabetic), the existence of such an excess is not absolute proof of diabetes. It is more usual to be sent for a blood glucose test. This blood will be taken from a vein, not a finger prick. By the time blood reaches the finger through the small blood vessels or capillaries, it has used up some of the glucose it was originally carrying so does not give an accurate picture. So it is important to measure the glucose in blood taken from a vein (the venous plasma glucose concentration). The normal glucose concentration that you would expect to find, according to World Health Organization (WHO) criteria, is below 7.8 millimols per litre.

A diabetic, according to the WHO criteria, is one whose "venous plasma glucose concentration" when they have been fasting, remains at 7.8mmol/litre, but rises to above 11.1mmol/litre on a random blood sample. Between "normal" and "diabetic" they list a third category of those with "impaired glucose tolerance" (7.8mmol/litre fasting and between 7.8 and 11.1mmol/litre on a random test). These people may return to normal, may go on to develop full-blown diabetes or remain at the same level. They should, however, follow a diabetic regime and keep themselves as healthy as possible.

TREATMENT

Although serious, even IDDM has become a treatable condition following the arrival of injectable insulin. Provided you are prepared to stick to your regime, there is no reason why you should not lead a full life.

The key to the management and treatment of both IDDM and NIDDM is to take over the job normally performed by the insulin in the body and keep your blood sugar levels normal. Allowing them to get too high, or too low, can cause a variety of problems and is to be avoided. This does not mean getting paranoid about blood sugar levels or diet – merely keeping a sensible watch on both.

For NIDDMs a change in diet, possibly in conjunction with medication to lower blood glucose levels, will frequently achieve the desired result. Indeed, changes to the diet may improve the health of an individual to such an extent that the onset of their diabetes may be viewed as something of a blessing.

IDDMs have benefited from the development of sophisticated blood testing techniques. These usually involve taking a drop of blood from the finger or ear lobe and have made it much easier to control blood glucose levels, either by changing the diet or the insulin dose.

Whether you have been diagnosed as being an insulin dependent diabetic or a diabetic who is non insulin dependent, your doctor will instruct you in the use of your drugs, insulin and glucose testing equipment. He or she will also give you dietary guidance or send you to a dietitian. The principles and practices for a good diabetic diet are described later in this introduction and further amplified in the recipe section.

SYMPTOMS

Thirst (polydipsia) and passing large quantities of urine (polyuria)
If the levels of glucose in the blood are too high, the kidneys no longer filter all the glucose and some escapes into the urine. The extra glucose thickens the urine, it draws extra water with it to help it to flow through the kidneys, and this causes the bladder to fill. The individual needs to urinate often and in copious amounts. At the same time the body becomes dehydrated, which leads to a terrible thirst.

Constipation
As the body becomes more dehydrated, constipation becomes almost inevitable.

Tiredness and weight loss
Since our bodies acquire their energy from glucose, anyone whose body cannot access the glucose circulating in the blood will be short of energy and therefore tired. In an effort to replace this energy, the body will break down other cells/body tissues thus causing a weight loss that can be dramatic.

Blurred vision
Excess sugar in the blood makes it thick and syrupy. In some diabetics, this can upset the focusing of the eyes – their vision becomes blurred.

Infections
When the blood becomes thick and syrupy due to the presence of excess glucose, this may also effect the functioning of the immune system. The undiagnosed diabetic may be prone to all kinds of infections, including skin eruptions, urinary tract infections, such as thrush or cystitis, and chest infections.

Pins and needles
Changes in the blood glucose levels may also affect nerve functions, resulting in tingling or pins and needles in the hands or feet.

ALTERNATIVE THERAPIES

Once the pancreas has given up on insulin production, it can very rarely be "kicked back into action". However, certain alternative or complementary therapies can stimulate pancreatic function, improve the body's insulin response and moderate glucose levels, so they are worth considering both in cases of non insulin dependent diabetes and in the immediate aftermath of the onset of insulin dependent diabetes, when there may still be some residual function in the pancreas.

Equally important is the diabetic's need to keep as fit and healthy – in both mind and body – as possible. It is recognized that stress does more damage to our health than almost anything else – and that many alternative therapies are very helpful in dealing with stress. Yoga, meditation, reflexology, aromatherapy and massage are the best-known stress relievers, but many people find spiritual healers, colour therapists or practising T'ai Chi just as helpful.

CHINESE MEDICINE

The Chinese have recognized diabetes as a disease for many thousands of years. However, Chinese medicine approaches the body, bodily functions and bodily malfunctions from an entirely different angle from Western medicine. To a Chinese doctor, diabetes is a sign of disharmony in the body, whose symptoms appear in the upper body (raging thirst, dry mouth, drinking huge quantities), middle body (large appetite and excessive eating accompanied by weight loss and constipation) and lower body (copious urination, progressive weight loss, etc).

Chinese medical treatment would therefore concentrate on restoring the harmony within the individual with the aim of improving the symptoms and addressing the disease.

Even if this approach does not directly affect insulin production or control, improving the body's natural harmony should improve the diabetic's general health and therefore their ability to cope well with diabetes. However, insulin dependent diabetics must not change their insulin regime if they attend a Chinese physician, except on the express instruction of their diabetes specialist.

RELAXATION AND MASSAGE THERAPIES

It is recognized that stress plays a significant role in the development of diabetes. Any therapy that reduces stress and helps you to relax is therefore likely to have a beneficial effect upon control of your diabetes and your general health.

Yoga and meditation have been found to have a positive impact on blood glucose levels, while moderate exercise helps insulin to work more efficiently in the body.

Reflexology helps to tone and relax the body and, although it cannot address the cause of diabetes, it can alleviate some of the side effects.

Left: Yoga and meditation are both said to reduce blood glucose levels by helping you to relax and reduce stress.

SELF MASSAGE

Aromatherapy (massage with essential herbal oils) is not only relaxing, but can also improve circulation and therefore help to heal the leg and foot ulcers to which some diabetics are prone.

The therapeutic potential of aromatherapy oils, although recognized in the past, has been largely ignored until recently. However, it is now realized that concentrated oils (made from plants and herbs that filled our ancestors' medicine chests) can be very helpful for many specific complaints.

Essential oils are easily absorbed through the skin into the bloodstream and so are particularly effective for circulatory problems. Some oils, such as hyssop, are good for the circulation as a whole; others, such as grapefruit, lemon, lime, fennel and white birch, are lymphatic stimulants; while spike lavender, rosemary, eucalyptus, peppermint and thyme stimulate sluggish circulation. Massage is a good way to apply essential oils as it is relaxing, and it also ensures that the oils are effectively absorbed.

LEG AND FOOT MASSAGE

Self-massage is relatively easy and can help considerably in reducing stiffness and sluggishness of blood flow in the legs.

1 Start a leg massage by working on the thighs, so that any fluid in the calves will have somewhere to go as the upper leg relaxes. Using both hands, knead one thigh at a time, by squeezing between the fingers and thumb.

2 Squeeze with each hand alternately for the best effect, working from the knee to the hip and back. Repeat on the other thigh.

3 Around the knees, do a similar kneading action but just using the fingers for a lighter effect and working in smaller circles.

4 Bend your leg, and if possible raise the foot on to a chair or handy ledge. With your thumbs, work on the back of each calf with a circular, kneading action. Repeat this action a few times on each leg, each time working from the ankle up to the knee.

5 Squeeze the foot with your hands, loosening up the muscles and gently stretching the arch.

6 To complete the massage, use firm pressure with your thumb to stretch the foot. Repeat on the other foot.

FOOD AND HERBAL MEDICINES

Certain foods and herbs, although they cannot reinstate pancreatic function, can help the pancreas to function more efficiently. They may also improve the absorption of insulin and lead to better control of glucose levels in the blood by the body and to improved circulation. This may, in part, be due to the nutrients found in these foods and herbs (see Nutritional Medicine below), but there is increasing evidence that certain foods and herbs have special health-giving properties, which cannot be entirely attributed to their vitamin or mineral content.

FOODS WITH HEALTH-GIVING PROPERTIES

- Whole oats, onions, globe artichokes and pulses all have the ability to reduce blood sugar.
- Wheat germ, underripe bananas, turkey, fish, walnuts, red peppers and cruciferous vegetables, such as broccoli and cauliflower (all good sources of Vitamin B6), help to control blood sugar levels.
- Shellfish, lean meat, wholegrain cereals, pulses, pumpkin seeds and nuts are all high in chromium and zinc (diabetics are commonly deficient in both minerals).
- Bilberries have been found to help in the control of diabetic retinopathy.
- Wheatgerm, sunflower seeds, rapeseed oils, almonds and sweet potatoes (all containing high levels of Vitamin E) have been shown to help improve diabetic circulation and neuropathy.
- Fresh nettle juice has been used since Roman times to stimulate the circulation, while dandelions have an equally lengthy pedigree for the stimulation of the liver (where glucose is stored).

Above: Dandelions have been used for years as a stimulant for the liver.

NUTRITIONAL MEDICINE

Effects of nutrient deficiencies

Although it has long been recognized that we need a wide range of vitamins and minerals for our bodies to function efficiently, there is a growing belief that many of today's degenerative illnesses, such as diabetes, could be caused by serious deficiencies in micronutrients, such as vitamins, minerals and amino acids. These deficiencies, it is argued, have resulted from our eating over-processed foods, living in a highly polluted environment and subjecting ourselves to hitherto unknown levels of stress. Research is going on all the time and continues to reveal links between certain degenerative conditions and particular nutrient deficiencies.

Chromium is an essential trace element. Although it is only present in minute quantities in the body, it appears to be necessary for blood sugar control and the proper action of insulin. Unfortunately chromium is removed from refined carbohydrates during processing. Chromium is difficult to take as a supplement but is absorbed from brewer's yeast, black pepper, calf's liver, wheat germ, wholemeal bread and cheese.

Vitamins B6 and B12 can both help blood sugar control. Vitamin B12 levels can be reduced by certain diabetic drugs, so it is useful to include sources of this vitamin (lean meat and dairy produce) in the diet.

Above: Nutritional supplements can help to ensure that you are getting the right amounts of some vitamins, minerals and essential fatty acids.

Vitamin C is known to strengthen fragile blood capillaries, especially in the eye, and to reduce elevated cholesterol levels – both conditions that affect diabetics.

Zinc, magnesium and potassium are all very important for diabetics, but levels can be seriously depleted through excess urination. Zinc is important for combating infections such as eczema, acne and thrush, many of which afflict diabetics. Magnesium is also important for the proper functioning of the kidneys.

Essential fatty acids There is increasing evidence that a diabetic's absorption of essential fatty acids may be impeded by raised blood sugar or insulin deficiency so taking a supplement, such as Evening Primrose oil, may help prevent diabetic complications.

KEEPING BLOOD GLUCOSE LEVELS NORMAL

The ideal state for a diabetic is for blood sugar levels to remain normal. Careful monitoring of these, a good diet and medication where necessary are basic strategies. However, many other aspects of the diabetic's life may impinge on his or her blood sugar levels.

BLOOD GLUCOSE LEVELS

Changing exercise levels, for example, can affect both the efficiency of insulin uptake and the rate at which the sugar in the blood is used up. Stress of any kind may cause adrenalin release that will increase the level of sugar in the blood. Infections, injuries or operations are seen by the body as stress. The body reacts by releasing adrenalin or other hormones into the bloodstream, and these again push up the sugar levels. Pregnancy causes changes in blood sugar levels, as do monthly periods and the menopause. Medical drugs, especially steroids and some diuretics and anti-depressants, can also affect blood sugar levels. If any of these factors apply, it is essential to monitor your blood sugar levels even more carefully than usual, adapting your diet or adjusting your insulin dose or the levels of the drug you take to lower blood glucose, in consultation with your doctor, if necessary.

Serious fluctuations in glucose levels cause hypoglycaemia (too little sugar) and hyperglycaemia (too much sugar) and have very specific symptoms, which need to be treated immediately. If dramatic rises (and, more especially, falls) in blood sugar are treated immediately, there are unlikely to be long-term effects. However, persistent slightly raised blood sugar levels of about 8–19mmol/litre do have a number of serious consequences in terms of health.

CORONARY HEART DISEASE

Elevated triglycerides (fats in the blood) are a common feature of poorly controlled diabetes and add greatly to the risk of coronary heart disease (when the arteries supplying blood to the heart "fur up", thus depriving the heart muscle of the blood it needs to function properly), so diabetics need to be particularly careful about eating a low-fat diet and ensuring that they are not overweight.

STROKE

High blood pressure is another area which diabetics need to watch. Keeping their weight normal, stopping smoking and eating a low-fat, low-salt diet will usually help a great deal to minimize the risk of strokes.

Below: Pregnancy will affect blood glucose levels, which need to be monitored.

NEUROPATHY

Diabetic neuropathy is very common in long-term and poorly controlled diabetics. Although there are many variations, neuropathy happens when the nerve ends become damaged (as a result of excess glucose flowing through the capillaries or small veins). Neuropathy normally affects the hands and feet (tingling or pins and needles in the hands and feet is one of the symptoms of diabetes) and can, over a period, result in loss of all feeling in the extremities.

Left: Exercise, such as jogging, increases the rate at which sugar in the blood is used up – to prevent a dangerous dip in your blood glucose level, eat a small carbohydrate snack before, or straight after, any exercise.

Neuropathy presents two problems. One is that the circulation to the more remote areas of the body gets worse and this can lead to infected wounds, bad healing and, in the worst cases, gangrene. Feet and legs are especially prone to damage and need to be looked after and monitored with great care. The other problem is that the feet lose all sensation. This not only affects balance and the ability to walk properly but also means that the sufferer is at risk of injury, perhaps by being scalded by getting into too hot a bath, because their feet have become so insensitive to temperature.

Diabetics can also suffer some damage to their "autonomic nerves". These are the nerves that carry the instructions to the various organs, such as heart, kidneys, bladder and bowels, and tell them what to do. Damage to these autonomic nerves can result in poor bowel or bladder control, failure of the stomach to empty properly and similar problems. Normally all these functions will return to normal when the blood glucose levels are also returned to normal.

KIDNEY AND EYE DAMAGE

The kidneys and the eyes are two areas of the body filled with capillaries or tiny blood vessels that are especially prone to diabetic damage. Excess blood sugar can "clog" up both areas, but whereas kidney damage may be reversed or at least controlled by diet and good blood glucose control, damage to the eyes may be irreversible. Maintaining good control of blood glucose levels will minimize the damage. It is particularly important that diabetics have very regular eye checks and that these should include examination of the retina.

SKIN PROBLEMS

Because raised blood sugar makes one more prone to infection, especially skin infection, badly controlled diabetes will often result in boils, pimples, spots and rashes. Most of these will respond well to good diet and improved control.

This disturbing list of symptoms may sound like a life sentence, but diabetics should remember that most of them only occur when they do not look after themselves. These days, a diabetic diet is almost identical to the healthy diet recommended for all of us – so the diabetic should not be singled out as an oddity. Because of the huge improvement in both monitoring and injection techniques, even insulin dependent diabetics can check their blood sugar levels and administer their insulin both quickly and discreetly. However, this does not mean that you should keep your diabetes a secret. For a start, there is no reason to as you can live a perfectly full life with diabetes. Secondly, friends, colleagues and even strangers need to know that you are diabetic in case you should suffer a hyper- or hypoglycaemic attack. This is easily dealt with, but very frightening if you or others do not know what is going on. Consider wearing a diabetic bracelet or tag.

All diabetes does require is that you take it seriously and are organized about dealing with it. You must be rigorous about checking your glucose levels, you must always make sure that you have your insulin or drugs available and you must always ensure that you have extra glucose or carbohydrate food should you need it. Finally, you must be aware that your body is more sensitive to change than that of someone without diabetes so you must pay attention to what it tells you in terms of "feeling different" or unwell. Your body is the best possible monitor of its own condition, so it is important to listen to it!

HYPER- AND HYPOGLYCAEMIA

Hyper- and hypoglycaemia occur when blood sugar levels rise too high (hyper) or fall too low (hypo).

HYPERGLYCAEMIA

The symptoms of hyperglycaemia are usually less dramatic than those of hypoglycaemia, but because tissue damage may result if the blood sugar levels remain too high (usually over 11–12mmol/litre), it is important to get the levels down quickly.

Elevated levels of blood sugar can be the result of uncontrolled long-term diabetes, but there can also be more immediate causes. Forgetting to take your insulin or blood glucose drugs will cause your blood sugar levels to rise, as will eating much more than you usually do – or eating a fattier or more sugary meal than normal.

Reducing the amount of exercise you usually take could affect glucose levels. An infection, illness, operation or accident could all cause blood sugar levels to rise, as can pregnancy and menstruation. Careful monitoring will reveal the raised levels quickly – anything over 11mmol/litre is undesirable – and changes in insulin, drugs or diet should get you back to normal.

HYPOGLYCAEMIA

Hypoglycaemia can occur in non-diabetics whose blood sugar levels fall too low; the official definition is below 2.5mmol/litre. However, this reaction is most frequently seen in diabetics who have taken more insulin than they need or eaten too little – or exercised too much – relative to their last dose of insulin or glucose-lowering drugs.

Although the symptoms of hypoglycaemia can be dramatic, its results are seldom serious, and it is extremely easy to treat. All you need is a rapid intake of sugar in the form of glucose tablets (Dextrose, Dextro), sugar lumps, honey, candy, fruit juice or sweet biscuits. Even when the symptoms are quite extreme, the diabetic will be back to normal in a matter of minutes.

Above: Glucose tablets are a simple and speedy remedy to mild hypoglycaemia.

However, they then need to back up the instant injection of glucose with more solid food, as the excess insulin will quickly absorb the initial blast of glucose and will need something further to work on.

The problem with hypoglycaemia is that the brain is utterly dependent on an adequate supply of glucose to function properly. The first sign that a diabetic is suffering from a "hypo" may be a failure in his or her logical reasoning powers. This can manifest itself as a refusal to accept that they may be suffering from a hypo – which is why it is particularly important for friends and colleagues to know that they are diabetic (and for the diabetic to carry a card or consider wearing an identifying bracelet or badge), so that if their hypo symptoms take the form of denial, someone else can get a glucose tablet into their mouth.

Hypo symptoms vary enormously, but they often include lack of concentration, difficulty in making even simple decisions or a feeling of being muddled. A common feeling is that you must finish whatever you are doing, even though you are feeling odd. This is particularly dangerous if you are driving a car, so diabetics must make every effort to recognize and combat this compulsion.

Hypos can often cause behavioural changes and quite violent mood swings. Coordination may also be impaired. They may stagger as if drunk and have difficulty in performing the simplest task – like unwrapping a glucose tablet!

If unrecognized and untreated, a hypo will eventually cause a diabetic to lose consciousness, but even then an injection of glucagon (the antidote to insulin) will bring the diabetic round to the point where they can be fed a proper dose of glucose.

Since symptoms are so varied, it is important that diabetics are aware of changes in their physical or mental states, that they monitor their blood sugar levels regularly, compensate for any changes in their daily routine and always carry glucose tablets (or the equivalent) with them. Long-term diabetics should be aware that over time symptoms of hypo decrease so that their blood sugar may fall without them having any symptoms at all.

A FEW WORDS OF WARNING

- Ignore rising blood sugar levels at your peril. Your body's reaction will not be as rapid as with low levels, but if ignored rising blood sugar levels can put you into a coma.
- Never give up your insulin or drug regime – even if you are vomiting. The greater the stress on the body, the greater its need for insulin to combat rising blood sugar levels. Vomiting is serious for a diabetic, so maintain your drug regime and consult a doctor.
- Because the body is infinitely adaptable, some people will feel quite ill when their blood sugar is only slightly raised, while others will still feel relatively okay with seriously high levels. Moreover, long-term undiagnosed diabetics may have got used to having high levels of sugar in their blood so they will not even notice feeling ill.
- It is particularly important to monitor your blood sugar levels on a regular basis, even if you feel fine.

HEALTHY EATING

Diet is the backbone of both insulin dependent and non insulin dependent diabetic management, and the first line of attack in stabilizing blood sugar control. Today, the diabetic diet varies little from the diet that everyone should be eating: to eat at least five portions of fruit and vegetables each day, to take in less than 30 per cent of calories from fat (with most of it coming from mono- and polyunsaturated fats), to reduce the intake of salt (sodium) and sweet foods and to eat plenty of fibre.

THE "OLD" APPROACH

Because sugar is derived from carbohydrates, when the mechanism of carbohydrate absorption was less well understood than it is today, it was thought that diabetics should avoid all carbohydrates. This meant that they had to live on a high-protein, high-fat diet and suffer the side-effects, such as high blood pressure, now associated with such a diet. Moreover, a high-fat diet caused them to gain weight.

Below: Protein is needed for growth and cell repair – wholegrain rice, beans, lentils, tofu and walnuts are all good sources.

TODAY'S APPROACH

Research over the last 25 years has turned this thinking on its head, and, although present-day diabetics still have to monitor their diet and their carbohydrate intake fairly carefully, they are now encouraged to eat plenty of the right kind of carbohydrate foods, while even a small amount of sugar as such is no longer entirely out of the question.

The food that we eat is made up of proteins, fats, carbohydrates, fibre, micronutrients (vitamins and minerals) and water. The last four (fibre, vitamins, minerals and water) are all essential for the proper functioning of the body but they do not provide us with energy as such (measured in kilo-calories or kilo-joules). This we need to get from proteins, fats and carbohydrates.

PROTEINS

Proteins (found in pulses, peas and beans, soya products, such as tofu, nuts, cereals, meat, fish and dairy products, such as cheese, milk and cream) are essential for growth in children and for cell repair in adults. We need to get up to 20 per cent of our daily energy intake in the form of proteins.

FATS

Fats (found primarily in meat and dairy products, but also in vegetable and fish oils and nuts) are essential to the proper functioning of the body. However, we need the right kind of fat and the right amount. The average Western diet contains far too much of the "wrong" kind of fat – saturated – which leads to obesity, heart problems and strokes. The recommended maximum number of daily calories which should come from fat is between 30 and 35 per cent. Unfortunately many Westerners obtain well over 40 per cent of their calories from fat.

Fats are broken down into saturated fats (mainly from the fat on meat, but also dairy products, such as cream, full-fat milk, butter and cheese, and nuts), polyunsaturated fats and mono-unsaturated fats (from vegetable oils such as olive oil and sunflower oil and from fish oils).

The subject of fats is a very complex one, but for the purposes of the diabetic diet the main thing to

Above: Sunflower oil (left) contains mostly polyunsaturated fats, while olive oil is made up of mainly monounsaturated fats.

remember is that saturated fats are to be avoided. These are more likely to cause excess cholesterol to be deposited in the arteries and, because they are higher in calories, obesity is a likely outcome. Diabetics may have high fat concentrations in their blood anyhow (making them more vulnerable to arteriosclerosis), so they should avoid making these levels even higher.

Above: Many different foods, such as (clockwise from top right) milk, pistachio nuts, butter, almonds, cream and cheese, contain fats. Dairy products, such as cheese, butter and milk are sources of saturated fats, which should be avoided by diabetics, while foods such as nuts are good sources of polyunsaturated fats, which, like monoun-saturated fats are much more beneficial.

CARBOHYDRATES

Carbohydrates (known in "diet-speak" as CHOs) also come in different guises – simple and complex carbohydrates.

Simple (refined or sugary) carbohydrates consist of various forms of what we know broadly as sugar or sucrose. In fact, sucrose is made up from glucose and fructose (fruit sugar). Both are essential for providing us with energy, but glucose is particularly important as the brain depends upon it to function efficiently.

Complex carbohydrates (unrefined carbohydrates) are to be found in starchy foods such as pulses (beans), oats, rice, potatoes and bread. Complex carbohydrates are made up of simple carbohydrates, glucose (see above) and fibres. These fibres may be soluble or insoluble. Soluble fibre is found in pulses, beans and legumes; it breaks down into a sort of gluey solution, which contains the carbohydrate. Insoluble fibre, such as that found in bran and such vegetables as celery and cabbage, has no nutritional value but is used by the body to move food through the system and to push out what is not wanted as waste.

Once they enter the digestive system, complex carbohydrates are broken down by the digestive juices into their components parts – sucrose and fibre. For a diabetic, the virtue of a carbohydrate made up of sucrose and soluble fibre (pulses, peas and beans) is that the gluey solution into which the soluble fibre turns prevents the system from absorbing the glucose too fast, thus giving the diabetic's impaired glucose handling system more time to absorb it. The disadvantage of simple carbohydrates (sugar or sucrose) is that they are absorbed almost immediately into the bloodstream, causing sudden glucose "peaks".

Although studies suggest that if it is eaten along with lots of starchy, high-fibre carbohydrate, a small amount of pure sugar can be successfully absorbed by some diabetics without creating glucose peaks, medical advice would still be to avoid sugar whenever possible. "Sugar" in this context would include sugar itself (in tea or coffee etc), sweets and candies, jams and jellies, cake and biscuits sweetened with sugar or fructose, and sweetened fizzy drinks.

"DIABETIC" FOODS

Medical advice is also to avoid expensive proprietary diabetic foods. Although their actual sucrose content may be lower than that of the foods they are meant to replace, they may use fructose or sorbitol as sweeteners (there is little medical evidence that fructose is any better for diabetics than glucose, and sorbitol can cause bowel problems if eaten in large quantities). Finally, these foods may make up for their low-sugar content by having a high-fat content!

Below: Unrefined or complex carbohydrates, which are found in such foods as (clockwise from top right) wholemeal bread, potatoes, oats, haricot beans, rice and lentils, are absorbed more slowly into the bloodstream.

THE DIABETIC'S DAY-TO-DAY DIET

The first thing that the diabetic must remember is that, because the body's ability to absorb sugar is impaired, the system must never be "overloaded". In practice, this means that he or she should have three regularly spaced, moderately sized meals, usually breakfast, lunch and dinner, with two or three regular snacks in between, such as elevenses, mid-afternoon tea and a snack at bed time. For an insulin dependent diabetic the meals must be timed to come 15–30 minutes after the insulin injection so that the insulin has had time to be absorbed into the bloodstream and is ready to cope with the food.

If you are a newly diagnosed diabetic and have led a rather disorganized life you may find forcing yourself to stick to specific times for meals difficult, but it will prove worth it. And you can console yourself with the thought that if the rest of us ate on a more regular basis we would all feel a lot better too!

BALANCE

A diabetic should try to ensure that each meal or snack is balanced to include proteins, fats and carbohydrates. This is not difficult to achieve, as many snacks naturally contain all three components in varying amounts. A ham sandwich, for example, includes protein (ham), fat (butter, spread) and carbohydrate (bread).

It is important that the diabetic does not miss out on any one element, especially the carbohydrate. Diabetics used to be given a list of what were known as "carbohydrate exchanges", which allocated a carbohydrate value to each food. They then had to work out how much carbohydrate was in each meal they ate, allocate their meal allowance of carbohydrate and devise a "swap" system if they wanted to change any element of this diet. Today, although diabetic practitioners still allot a total carbohydrate allowance to be spread over the day (based on the diabetic's own lifestyle, eating patterns, medication, etc), this does not need to be as rigid as the old exchange system.

AVOIDING EXCESSIVE CALORIE INTAKE

Whereas insulin dependent diabetics are often very thin, non insulin diabetics, especially long-term ones, tend to obesity – partly of course because the traditional diabetic diet was high in fat and protein. However, it is really important for diabetics to keep their weight down so as to minimize circulatory and other diseases.

As anyone knows who has tried to diet, the only long-term answer is to reduce the total amount of food that you eat and change the nature of that food.

Reducing the amount of sugar in your diet will set you well on the way; reducing the amount of fat, especially saturated fat, in your diet will help even more. And reduction does not necessarily mean total deprivation!

Right: Fizzy, sweetened drinks, full-sugar jam, sweet biscuits, confectionery, chocolate and cakes aren't completely banned, but consumption of these high-calorie foods should be kept to a minimum.

REDUCING SUGAR

Most diabetic practitioners would prefer their patients to stop sweetening their tea and coffee. However, if the thought is too terrible to contemplate, intense sweeteners, such as Aspartame (NutraSweet, Canderel) or Saccharin (Sweet'n'Low, Hermesetas) are better than sugar, but their consumption should be kept to a minimum.

Sugar in drinks other than coffee and tea – fizzy drinks, colas, etc – should be avoided. Not only do these fizzy drinks give an instant glucose hit (bad for diabetic control), but they are also very calorific (the average cola contains the equivalent of seven teaspoons of sugar). Fizzy water or fresh fruit juice diluted with water are preferred – or, if desperate, the diabetic should stick with low-calorie artificially sweetened, fizzy drinks.

Sugar in baking can almost always be replaced with dried or fresh fruits, as is amply illustrated in the recipes that follow. Although fruit contains fructose, this is buried in fibrous flesh, so it is absorbed much more slowly into the system. Fruit also gives a far better flavour to cakes and desserts than granulated sugar, which may be sweet but has no flavour of its own.

Diabetics, indeed all dieters, should also scrutinize labels for added sugar.

Below: Avoid sweetened drinks and opt instead for fizzy water or fresh fruit juice diluted with water.

Sometimes this is easy to avoid – buy fruits canned in fruit juice instead of syrup, for example – but it is not always that clear. Remember that on an ingredients list sucrose, fructose, glucose, maltose, honey, lactose, malt and invert corn syrup are all sugar, under different names.

Sweets and chocolate bars are to be avoided except as a snack before or after sport. Like the fizzy drinks, these not only deliver an instant glucose "hit", but they are very high in calories. If total deprivation is not to be borne, try buying chocolate, for example, in thin tablets or drops. It is amazing how satisfying even a morsel of chocolate can be if you nibble it rather than wolfing down a whole bar!

If an apple does not fill that sweet gap, try a few raisins or fresh dates.

They are just as sweet as a mint or a bar of chocolate but the sugar they contain is embedded in fibre.

Below: To avoid sugar, choose fruits canned in fruit juice, and try apples, fresh dates and raisins as an alternative snack.

REDUCING FATS

Reducing the amount of calories from fat – especially saturated fat – will help greatly in overall weight control and will also fit in with the specifically diabetic diet. Again, it need not be that difficult to achieve: Some of the new low-fat spreads are really very palatable and work excellently in pastry and baking. Does one always need butter or a spread? A ham sandwich with mustard needs neither; a cheese sandwich tastes as good, if not better, with a little low-fat mayonnaise and a lettuce leaf as it does with a thick layer of butter.

Use extra virgin olive oil or sunflower oil, not butter or lard, for cooking – and try not to use even that. Meat and vegetables for stews do not need to be fried at the start of cooking. If they are cooked long and slowly enough, they will have plenty of flavour. If the occasional plate of chips is a must, use the oven-ready ones, which have a substantially lower fat content. Ideally the chips should be abandoned in favour of a baked potato – but a baked potato filled with canned tuna and sweetcorn, or canned salmon

or baked beans, not with piles of butter or cheese!

Like chips, crisps should really be on the forbidden list. Not only are they calorific and high in fat (even the low-fat ones), but they are very salty – and everyone should be reducing their salt intake! Nuts or (even better) seeds, such as sunflower or pumpkin, maybe lightly salted, are just as good with a drink or as a snack and are very much more nutritious.

Above: Choose a low-fat filling for baked potatoes: here the potatoes are simply spiced with curry-flavoured onions and served topped with a generous dollop of low-fat natural yogurt.

USING WHOLEMEAL BREADS AND FLOURS

Even devoted white bread fans, if they persevere with wholemeal breads, will find that although wholemeal breads are not as soft, they have much more flavour. The same applies to using wholemeal flour in baking. The pastry may not be quite as light, but it will be much more flavoursome. There are several other flours that can be used for "lighter but healthier" baking, the most successful of which is gram or chick-pea flour. This is used a lot in Indian cooking. For a diabetic, it has the advantage of being made from a pulse, so it is filled with soluble fibre. Gram flour can be substituted for white flour in most instances and, although the pastry will be a little crumbly, it will taste delicious.

Left: Wholemeal bread is a healthier option than white bread. However, olive-oil breads, such as ciabatta, flavoured with olives or sun-dried tomatoes, are better than highly processed sliced white breads.

FILLING YOURSELF UP

The best way to prevent yourself nibbling – or having the urge to nibble – is by filling yourself up! Try eating large platefuls of colourful salad leaves and raw vegetables, such as tomatoes, peppers, cucumbers, carrots and radishes, or lightly cooked vegetables (most of which, being low in fat and carbohydrate, are on the "eat as much as your like" list for diabetics). For a main meal, bulk out vegetables and salads with cooked wholemeal rice, pasta or cooked beans and pep them up with plenty of chopped fresh herbs and a simple, tasty dressing made from lemon juice and extra virgin olive oil. It is amazing how satisfying they are. Because the food is full of fibre it will take some time for the body to digest, so that feeling of fullness will not have worn off within half an hour as it so often does after over-indulging on sticky cakes.

MONITORING FAT, SODIUM AND FIBRE INTAKES

Diabetics who do not need to lose weight still need to monitor their fat, sodium (salt) and fibre intakes. It is very important that diabetics keep the cholesterol levels in their blood under control to limit the risk of coronary heart disease. They should also keep their blood pressure down. A healthy, low-fat, low-salt, high-fibre diet will do all of these things.

Above: This pilaff of cooked wholemeal rice combined with plenty of lightly cooked vegetables and prawns is a good example of a simple and satisfying – yet low-fat – meal.

TIPS FOR CUTTING CALORIES

• Using a slightly smaller plate so that a smaller portion still looks generous is an old, but very successful, trick!

• Chewing rather than gulping one's food is another. Some experts recommend up to 20 "chews" per mouthful, but even eight or nine will extend the eating period so that the food seems to go further.

• If the weight still refuses to come off, keep a food diary, in which all food consumed is written down.

• Don't con yourself into thinking that you are sticking to a diet, if you forget about the broken biscuit you ate because it fell out of the packet, the chunk of cheese you ate while grating a piece for a recipe, the half sausage the children had left on their plates or the lick of the jam spoon as it went into the washing up.

• Cutting out these few unnecessary calories may be all that it takes for the required amount of weight to be lost.

MODERATION

It is very easy, especially for a newly diagnosed diabetic, to get paranoid about his or her diet. This is not only unnecessary but is positively unhelpful: all this does is raise stress levels, and it is well recognized that stress is more debilitating for a diabetic than for anyone else.

FOODS TO EAT AND FOODS TO AVOID

It is very important for diabetics to keep their overall diet, but the occasional "fall from grace" is not likely to be catastrophic, especially if it can be compensated for at the next meal.

At first it may be hard to remember what is, and is not, allowed, but this will soon become second nature. Comparing calorie values is an easy way to monitor general food intake, but it is even more useful to memorize the following categories of foods as early as possible.

FREE FOODS

These can be eaten whenever and in whatever quantity you want.

- all green and leafy vegetables
- cruciferous vegetables (cauliflower, broccoli, turnip, cabbage, etc)
- salad vegetables (tomatoes, peppers, cucumbers, etc)
- all members of the onion family
- green peas and green beans
- mushrooms
- fruits, such as redcurrants, cranberries and loganberries
- tea, coffee, water, tomato juice (in moderation), clear soups

Left: Eat as much as you like – there's no restriction on the quantity of fresh green beans and peas that diabetics can eat.

Below: Fruits, such as (clockwise from top) pears, grapes, nectarines, raspberries and plums must be counted as part of a diabetic's daily carbohydrate allocation, but make ideal between-meal snacks as well as instant high-fibre desserts.

Above: Salad vegetables, such as fresh tomatoes, cucumbers and a variety of colourful peppers, can be eaten in whatever quantity you want – they are very low in sugar, fat and calories, yet are a good source of micronutrients.

GOOD CARBOHYDRATE/ PROTEIN FOODS

These are good for diabetics to eat, but must be counted as part of an overall carbohydrate and protein allocation.

- all pulses, beans and peas
- brown rice and wholemeal pasta
- oats, wholemeal flours, breads, unsweetened biscuits, etc
- all root vegetables
- all fresh fruits
- all canned fruits as long as canned in fruit juice, not syrup
- dried fruits
- high-fibre unsweetened breakfast cereals
- lean meats or meat products
- fresh and frozen fish
- low-fat cheese, skimmed milk, low-fat yogurts
- all soya products

Right: Soya beans and tofu are good foods for diabetics to eat, however, soya margarine, a healthy alternative to butter, is still a fat and should be used sparingly.

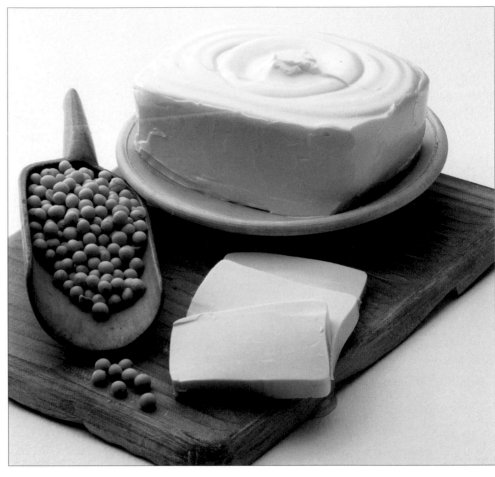

BORDERLINE FOODS

This list reflects less "good" carbohydrate foods and fatty foods – all right to have sometimes in specific quantities but not to overindulge in.

- white flour, bread, unsweetened biscuits, pastry, rice and pasta
- cornflour, arrowroot, semolina
- unsweetened breakfast cereals
- any fried potato products, such as chips and crisps
- full-fat cheese, cream, full-fat milk, yogurt
- fatty meats, including sausages
- salty meats and fish products
- fruit juices
- reduced-sugar jams, marmalade and other spreads
- alcohol

Left: Borderline foods, such as (clockwise from top) full-fat milk, full-fat, sweetened yogurts, full-fat cheeses and cream, can be eaten occasionally, but don't over-indulge!

BAD FOODS

These are to be avoided whenever possible and, when eaten, only to be consumed in very small quantities.

- sugar: caster, granulated, demerara; also honey and golden syrup
- sweets, such as candies, chocolate
- full-sugar chewing gum
- full-sugar jams, marmalades and similar spreads
- sweet biscuits, cakes and buns made with white flour and sugar
- desserts made with refined flours and refined sugar

- fruit canned in syrup
- ice cream and ice lollies
- fruit squashes, sweetened drinks, sweetened fizzy drinks and colas
- sweetened breakfast cereals

Below: No longer banned entirely, but sweet treats, such as (clockwise from top left) golden syrup, caster sugar, honey, icing sugar and demerara sugar should only be eaten in very small quantities.

Above: Chocolate biscuits, cakes and buns are best avoided by diabetics.

ALCOHOL

Alcohol, such as red wine and lager (*right*), is not entirely off limits for diabetics but must be taken in moderation and calculated into the diet. Beware of low-alcohol drinks. Because less of the sugar has been converted to alcohol, they may contain more sugar. Conversely, low-sugar drinks may contain more alcohol! Remember that alcohol is calorific; if you are trying to lose weight, keep your consumption low. It is also important to remember that excess alcohol consumption puts a strain on the liver and the pancreas – both organs that are already under pressure in a diabetic.

ABOUT THE RECIPES

We hope that the recipes in this collection will give diabetics (and non-diabetics) ideas for other dishes that will fulfil the diabetic diet criteria. Any good cookery book should encourage experimentation, so feel free to change – or indeed improve the recipes that follow.

Our aim has been to introduce ingredients high in soluble fibre, such as pulses and beans and low in fats and sugars, combined with other more familiar ingredients.

Many of the main course dishes add lentils or dried beans to meat and vegetables. The only oil in savoury dishes is olive oil or sunflower oil. All baking is done with low-fat spreads and natural fruit sweeteners (apart from the occasional chocolate treat). Those who have never cooked with dried or fresh fruit purées will be amazed how good the results are – and how little they miss the sugar.

Sodium Levels – Regular stock cubes can be very high in salt, so look out for "natural" or "organic" stock cubes with no added salt. Whenever possible, buy "no added salt or sugar" canned beans and vegetables.

STARTERS AND SOUPS

Vegetable starters and soups are ideal for diabetics as they are often low in fat and sugar and high in fibre. What is more, it is easy to make them appealing to the whole family. This colourful and tasty collection includes a delectable salad made with avocados and strawberries, tender courgettes stuffed with a piquant tomato and herb salsa, and a range of stunning soups made with vibrant vegetables and pulses.

Chilled Stuffed Courgettes

Full of flavour but low in calories and fat, this superb starter is also ideal as a light lunch dish.

INGREDIENTS

Serves 6
6 courgettes
1 Spanish onion, very finely chopped
1 garlic clove, crushed
60–90ml/4–6 tbsp well-flavoured
 French dressing
1 green pepper
3 tomatoes, peeled and seeded
15ml/1 tbsp rinsed capers
5ml/1 tsp chopped fresh parsley
5ml/1 tsp chopped fresh basil
sea salt and ground black pepper
parsley sprigs, to garnish

1 Top and tail the courgettes, but do not peel them. Bring a large shallow pan of lightly salted water to the boil, add the courgettes and simmer for 2–3 minutes until they are lightly cooked. Drain well.

2 Cut the courgettes in half lengthways. Carefully scoop out the flesh, leaving the courgette shells intact, and chop the flesh into small cubes. Place in a bowl and cover with half the chopped onion. Dot with the crushed garlic. Drizzle 30ml/2 tbsp of the dressing over, cover and marinate for 2–3 hours. Wrap the courgette shells tightly in clear film, and chill them until they are required.

3 Cut the pepper in half and remove the core and seeds. Dice the flesh. Chop the tomatoes and capers finely. Stir the pepper, tomatoes and capers into the courgette mixture, with the remaining onion and the chopped herbs. Season with salt and pepper. Pour over enough of the remaining dressing to moisten the mixture and toss well. Spoon the filling into the courgette shells, arrange on a platter and serve garnished with parsley.

--- NUTRITION NOTES ---

Per portion:	
Energy	95kcals/390kJ
Fat, total	7.3g
saturated fat	1.1g
polyunsaturated fat	0.9g
monounsaturated fat	4.9g
Carbohydrate	5.3g
sugar, total	4.75g
starch	0.2g
Fibre – NSP	1.95g
Sodium	60mg

Persian Omelette

Serve this spiced omelette hot or cold, in wedges as a starter, or cut it into bite-size pieces for serving with drinks. The herbs and nuts add texture and taste.

INGREDIENTS

Serves 8

30ml/2 tbsp olive oil or sunflower oil
2 leeks, finely chopped
350g/12oz fresh spinach, washed and
    chopped, or 150g/5oz thawed frozen
    chopped spinach, drained
12 eggs
8 spring onions, finely chopped
2 handfuls fresh parsley, finely chopped
1–2 handfuls fresh coriander, chopped
2 fresh tarragon sprigs, chopped, or
    2.5ml/½ tsp dried tarragon
handful of fresh chives, chopped
1 small fresh dill sprig, chopped, or
    1.5ml/¼ tsp dried dill
2–4 fresh mint sprigs, chopped
40g/1½oz/⅓ cup walnuts or pecan
    nuts, chopped
40g/1½oz/½ cup pine nuts
sea salt and ground black pepper
salad, to serve

1 Heat the oil in a large shallow pan that can be used under the grill. Add the leeks and fry them gently for about 5 minutes until they are just beginning to soften.

2 If using fresh spinach, add it to the pan containing the leeks and cook for 2–3 minutes over a medium heat until the spinach has just wilted.

3 Beat the eggs in a bowl with a fork. Add the leek and spinach mixture (or the leeks with the thawed frozen spinach), then stir in the spring onions, with all the herbs and nuts. Season with salt and pepper. Pour the mixture into the pan and cover with a lid or foil.

4 Cook over a very gentle heat for 25 minutes or until set. Remove the lid and brown the top under a hot grill. Serve, with salad.

NUTRITION NOTES

Per portion:
Energy	258kcals/1073kJ
Fat, total	21g
saturated fat	3.9g
polyunsaturated fat	6.1g
monounsaturated fat	8.7g
Carbohydrate	2.8g
sugar, total	2.3g
starch	0.15g
Fibre – NSP	1.9g
Sodium	192mg

Aubergine and Smoked Trout Pâté

INGREDIENTS

Serves 6
1 large aubergine
2–3 garlic cloves, unpeeled
4 smoked trout fillets
juice of 1 lemon
sea salt and ground black pepper
toast, to serve

—— NUTRITION NOTES ——

Per portion:

Energy	145kcals/609kJ
Fat, total	4.7g
saturated fat	1.05g
polyunsaturated fat	1.6g
monounsaturated fat	1.6g
Carbohydrate	1.6g
sugar, total	1.1g
starch	0.5g
Fibre – NSP	1.1g
Sodium	89mg

1 Slice the aubergine thickly and spread out the slices in a steamer. Tuck the whole garlic cloves among the slices. Steam over boiling water for 10–15 minutes until both the aubergine slices and the garlic cloves are quite soft.

2 Carefully cut the skins from around the aubergine slices using a small sharp knife.

3 Skin the trout fillets and chop them roughly. Put them in a food processor. Pop the garlic flesh out of the skins and add it to the processor with the aubergine slices. Add the lemon juice and process until smooth. Spoon into a bowl and season. Cool, then chill. Serve with toast.

Avocado and Strawberry Salad

The combination of avocado and strawberries works surprisingly well in this refreshing salad.

INGREDIENTS

Serves 6
2 large, ripe avocados
juice of 2–3 lemons
15 strawberries
120ml/4fl oz/½ cup low-fat
  natural yogurt
15–30 ml/1–2 tbsp chopped fresh mint
sea salt and ground black pepper
sprig of mint, to garnish

—— COOK'S TIP ——

Serve the salad straightaway, before the avocado slices have a chance to discolour.

1 Cut the avocados in half and remove the skin and stones. Cut the avocado flesh into thin slices, then place the slices in a bowl and sprinkle over half the lemon juice.

—— NUTRITION NOTES ——

Per portion:

Energy	93kcals/387kJ
Fat, total	8g
saturated fat	1.75g
polyunsaturated fat	0.9g
monounsaturated fat	4.9g
Carbohydrate	3.5g
sugar, total	2.8g
starch	0g
Fibre – NSP	1.5g
Sodium	20mg

2 Halve or slice the strawberries and toss them lightly with the avocado slices in the bowl. Mix the yogurt with enough cold water to give a pouring consistency. Stir in the mint and season to taste. Spoon the dressing over the salad, garnish with mint and serve.

Sweet Potato and Red Pepper Soup

As colourful as it is good to eat, this soup is a sure winner.

INGREDIENTS

Serves 6

500g/1¼lb sweet potato
2 red peppers, about 225g/8oz, seeded and cubed
1 onion, roughly chopped
2 large garlic cloves, roughly chopped
300ml/½ pint/1¼ cups dry white wine
1.2 litres/2 pints/5 cups vegetable or light chicken stock
Tabasco sauce (optional)
sea salt and ground black pepper
country bread, to serve

1 Peel the sweet potato and cut it into cubes. Put these in a saucepan with the red peppers, onion, garlic, wine and vegetable or chicken stock. Bring to the boil, lower the heat and simmer for 30 minutes or until all the vegetables are quite soft.

2 Transfer the mixture to a blender or food processor and process until smooth. Season to taste with salt, pepper and a generous dash of Tabasco, if liked. Pour into a tureen or serving bowl and cool slightly. Serve warm or at room temperature, with bread.

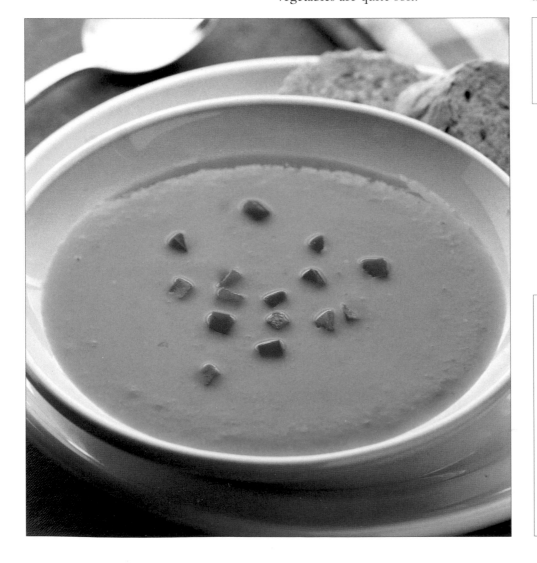

COOK'S TIP

Garnish the soup with finely diced red, green or yellow pepper, if you like.

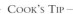

NUTRITION NOTES

Per portion:

Energy	122kcals/516kJ
Fat, total	0.4g
saturated fat	0.1g
polyunsaturated fat	0.17g
monounsaturated fat	0g
Carbohydrate	21.4g
sugar, total	7.9g
starch	13.2g
Fibre – NSP	2.8g
Sodium	37mg

Garlicky Lentil Soup

High in fibre, lentils make a very tasty soup. Unlike many pulses, they do not need to be soaked before being cooked.

INGREDIENTS

Serves 6

225g/8oz/1 cup red lentils, rinsed and drained
2 onions, finely chopped
2 large garlic cloves, finely chopped
1 carrot, very finely chopped
30ml/2 tbsp olive oil
2 bay leaves
generous pinch of dried marjoram or oregano
1.5 litres/2½ pints/6¼ cups vegetable stock
30ml/2 tbsp red wine vinegar
sea salt and ground black pepper
celery leaves, to garnish
crusty rolls, to serve

COOK'S TIP

If you buy your lentils loose, remember to tip them into a sieve or colander and pick them over, removing any pieces of grit, before rinsing them.

1 Put all the ingredients except the vinegar, garnish and seasoning in a large heavy-based saucepan. Bring to the boil over a medium heat, then lower the heat and simmer for 1½ hours, stirring the soup occasionally to prevent the lentils from sticking to the bottom of the pan.

2 Remove the bay leaves and add the red wine vinegar, with salt and pepper to taste. If the soup is too thick, thin it with a little extra vegetable stock or water. Serve the soup in heated bowls, garnished with celery leaves and accompanied by crusty rolls.

NUTRITION NOTES

Per portion:

Energy	167kcals/748kJ
Fat, total	5.6g
saturated fat	0.8g
polyunsaturated fat	0.65g
monounsaturated fat	3.7g
Carbohydrate	23.6g
sugar, total	2.6g
starch	19.3g
Fibre – NSP	2.45g
Sodium	18.5mg

Mrs Blencowe's Green Pea Soup with Spinach

This lovely green soup was invented by the wife of a seventeenth-century British Member of Parliament, and it has stood the test of time.

INGREDIENTS

Serves 6

450g/1lb/generous 3 cups podded fresh
   or frozen peas
1 leek, finely sliced
2 garlic cloves, crushed
2 rindless back bacon slices,
   finely diced
1.2 litres/2 pints/5 cups ham or
   chicken stock
30ml/2 tbsp olive oil
50g/2oz fresh spinach, shredded
40g/1½oz white cabbage, very
   finely shredded
½ small lettuce, very finely shredded
1 celery stick, finely chopped
large handful of parsley, finely chopped
½ carton mustard and cress
20ml/4 tsp chopped fresh mint
pinch of mace
sea salt and ground black pepper

1 Put the peas, leek, garlic and bacon in a large saucepan. Add the stock, bring to the boil, then lower the heat and simmer for 20 minutes.

2 About 5 minutes before the pea mixture is ready, heat the oil in a deep frying pan.

3 Add the spinach, cabbage, lettuce, celery and herbs. Cover and sweat the mixture over a low heat until soft.

COOK'S TIP

Use 25g/1oz frozen leaf spinach if fresh spinach is not available.

4 Transfer the pea mixture to a blender or food processor; process until smooth. Return to the clean saucepan, add the sweated vegetables and herbs and heat through. Season with mace, salt and pepper and serve.

--- NUTRITION NOTES ---

Per portion:	
Energy	140kcals/575kJ
Fat, total	7.6g
saturated fat	1.45g
polyunsaturated fat	1.2g
monounsaturated fat	4.4g
Carbohydrate	10g
sugar, total	2.7g
starch	5.8g
Fibre – NSP	4.4g
Sodium	165mg

Cream of Celeriac and Spinach Soup

Celeriac has a wonderful flavour
that is reminiscent of celery, but
also adds a slightly nutty taste.
Here it is combined with spinach
to make a delicious soup.

INGREDIENTS

Serves 6
1 leek
500g/1¼lb celeriac
1 litre/1¾ pints/4 cups water
250ml/8fl oz/1 cup dry white wine
200g/7oz fresh spinach leaves
semi-skimmed milk (optional)
25g/1oz/⅓ cup pine nuts
sea salt, ground black pepper and
    grated nutmeg

1 Trim and slit the leek. Rinse it
under running water to remove any
grit, then slice it thickly. Peel the
celeriac and dice the flesh.

2 Mix the water and wine in a jug.
Place the leek and celeriac, with
the spinach, in a deep saucepan and
pour over the liquid. Bring to the boil,
lower the heat and simmer for 10–15
minutes, until the vegetables are soft.

3 Purée the celeriac mixture, in
batches if necessary, in a blender or
food processor. Return to the clean
pan and season to taste with salt,
pepper and nutmeg. If the soup is too
thick, thin it with a little water or
semi-skimmed milk. Reheat gently.

4 Roast the pine nuts in a dry non-
stick frying pan until golden.
Sprinkle them over the soup and serve.

NUTRITION NOTES	
Per portion:	
Energy	82kcals/340kJ
Fat, total	3.5g
saturated fat	0.25g
polyunsaturated fat	1.9g
monounsaturated fat	0.85g
Carbohydrate	3.25g
sugar, total	2.7g
starch	0.5g
Fibre – NSP	4g
Sodium	124mg

FISH AND MEAT

Fish is excellent food for diabetics, and such dishes as a pilaff with spicy prawns, or parcels of filo pastry filled with sardines, are both healthy and light. Meat dishes, which need to be high in fibre for diabetics, tend to be heartier fare. The selection here includes beef and lentil balls cooked in a tomato sauce, leg of lamb roasted until tender with flageolet beans, and sausages combined with mixed beans and bacon to make a warming casserole.

Fennel and Smoked Haddock Chowder

This soup is substantial enough to serve as a main meal with plenty of poppy seed bread.

INGREDIENTS

Serves 8
1 large fennel bulb
2 large leeks, very finely sliced
225g/8oz new potatoes, scrubbed,
   halved or quartered if large
5ml/1 tsp dill seed
2 large garlic cloves, thinly sliced
½ lemon
1.5 litres/2½ pints/6¼ cups water
300ml/½ pint/1¼ cups dry
   white wine
225g/8oz smoked haddock
   fillet, skinned
sea salt and ground black pepper
chopped fresh parsley, to garnish

1 Quarter the fennel, cut away the core and slice each piece very finely. Place in a saucepan with the leeks, potatoes, dill seed and garlic. Cut the half lemon into thick slices and add these to the pan. Pour the water and wine into the pan.

2 Season with plenty of pepper, then bring to the boil, lower the heat and simmer for about 30 minutes or until the potatoes and fennel are both cooked through.

3 Cut the haddock into chunks, add to the pan and simmer the mixture for 10 minutes more. Remove the lemon slices. Stir the soup gently. Add salt and pepper to taste. Sprinkle with parsley and serve.

NUTRITION NOTES	
Per portion:	
Energy	75kcals/316kJ
Fat, total	0.5g
saturated fat	0.1g
polyunsaturated fat	0.15g
monounsaturated fat	0.1g
Carbohydrate	6g
sugar, total	1.5g
starch	4.35g
Fibre – NSP	1.2g
Sodium	221mg

Linguine with Smoked Salmon

INGREDIENTS

Serves 6

30ml/2 tbsp olive oil
115g/4oz/1 cup button mushrooms,
  finely sliced
250ml/8fl oz/1 cup dry white wine
7.5ml/1½ tsp fresh dill or 5ml/1 tsp
  dried dill weed
handful of fresh chives, snipped
300ml/½ pint/1¼ cups very low-fat
  unsweetened soya cream or very
  low-fat fromage frais
225g/8oz smoked salmon, cut into
  thin strips
lemon juice
350g/12oz fresh linguine or spaghetti
sea salt and ground black pepper
whole chives, to garnish

1 Heat the oil in a wide, shallow
saucepan. Add the finely sliced
mushrooms and fry them over a gentle
heat for 4–5 minutes until they are
softened but not coloured.

2 Pour the white wine into the pan.
Increase the heat and boil rapidly
for about 5 minutes, until the wine has
reduced considerably.

3 Stir in the herbs and the soya cream
or fromage frais. Fold in the salmon
and reheat gently, but do not let the
sauce boil or it will curdle. Stir in
pepper and lemon juice to taste. Cover
the pan and keep the sauce warm.

4 Cook the pasta in a large saucepan
of lightly salted boiling water until
just tender. Drain, rinse thoroughly in
boiling water and drain again. Turn
into a warmed serving dish and toss
gently with the salmon sauce before
serving, garnished with chives.

NUTRITION NOTES

Per portion:

Energy	346kcals/1464kJ
Fat, total	8.3g
saturated fat	1.35g
polyunsaturated fat	1.6g
monounsaturated fat	4.5g
Carbohydrate	42.4g
sugar, total	5.8g
starch	36.5g
Fibre – NSP	5.16g
Sodium	800mg

COOK'S TIP

Soya cream may be an acquired taste, but it
is a very successful low-fat substitute for
dairy cream in dishes like this one, with a
strong flavour of their own.

Sardine and Spinach Parcels

If you needed encouragement to eat more oily fish, this recipe will provide the perfect excuse.

INGREDIENTS

Serves 6

2 x 120g/4¼oz cans large sardines in oil
3 leeks, finely chopped
300g/11oz fresh spinach leaves, finely shredded
2 tomatoes, peeled, seeded and finely chopped
lemon juice
24 sheets of filo pastry, about 20cm/8in square, thawed if frozen
30ml/2 tbsp olive oil, for brushing filo
sea salt and ground black pepper
salad leaves, to garnish

1 Preheat the oven to 180°C/350°F/ Gas 4. Drain the oil from one of the cans of sardines into a frying pan. Set six sardines aside. Heat the oil and fry the leeks for 5 minutes. Add the spinach and tomatoes and cook over a low heat for 5 minutes until soft. Add salt, pepper and lemon juice to taste.

2 Stack four sheets of filo, brushing each sheet with olive oil and laying each sheet at an angle of 45° to the one below. Spoon a sixth of the vegetable mixture into the centre of the top sheet. Press a sardine into the middle of the vegetable mixture.

3 Fold over the filo to make a parcel, brushing each fold with olive oil. Brush the top of the parcel with oil and place it on a baking sheet. Make five more parcels. Bake the filo parcels for 20 minutes, or until the filo is crisp and brown. Garnish with salad leaves.

——— NUTRITION NOTES ———	
Per portion:	
Energy	251kcals/1048kJ
Fat, total	12g
saturated fat	1.9g
polyunsaturated fat	2.8g
monounsaturated fat	5.65g
Carbohydrate	22.5g
sugar, total	2.5g
starch	20g
Fibre – NSP	2.2g
Sodium	253mg

Turkish Prawn Pilaff

INGREDIENTS

Serves 6

60ml/4 tbsp olive oil
1 onion, finely chopped
2 large red peppers, seeded and finely
    chopped
2 garlic cloves, finely chopped
350g/12oz/1½ cups brown rice
5ml/1 tsp ground allspice
5ml/1 tsp ground cumin
10ml/2 tsp dried mint or basil
225g/8oz cooked peeled prawns,
    thawed if frozen
45ml/3 tbsp currants
juice of 2 large lemons
2 handfuls fresh parsley, finely chopped
sea salt and ground black pepper
salad, to serve

1 Heat the oil in a shallow saucepan. Fry the onion, peppers and garlic over a low heat for 10 minutes until the onion has softened but not browned.

NUTRITION NOTES

Per portion:

Energy	383kcals/1612kJ
Fat, total	12.6g
saturated fat	2g
polyunsaturated fat	1.7g
monounsaturated fat	7.9g
Carbohydrate	58g
sugar, total	10g
starch	47g
Fibre – NSP	2.4g
Sodium	606mg

2 Add the rice, spices and mint or basil. Stir over the heat for 2–3 minutes, then add enough water to cover the rice. Bring to the boil, lower the heat and simmer, uncovered, for 10–15 minutes or until the rice is just tender, but still has a little bite to it.

3 Add the prawns, currants and a little salt, to taste. Cook for about 4 minutes more, until the prawns have heated through, then add the lemon juice and chopped parsley. Add pepper to taste. Serve the pilaff warm or cold, with salad.

VEGETABLES AND VEGETARIAN DISHES

The increasing popularity of vegetarian food is good news for diabetics. Dishes, such as a casserole of red cabbage and apple, or baked vegetables with artichokes, can be served as main meals, or in smaller portions as accompaniments to meat or fish dishes. Others, such as a risotto made with red peppers and a flan of mushrooms and sunflower seeds, make excellent meals on their own, with a salad or served with another vegetable.

Red Cabbage and Apple Casserole

The brilliant colour and pungent flavour make this an excellent winter dish. Serve it solo, with plenty of rye bread, or as a vegetable accompaniment.

INGREDIENTS

Serves 6
3 onions, chopped
2 fennel bulbs, roughly chopped
675g/1½lb red cabbage, shredded
30ml/2 tbsp caraway seeds
3 large tart eating apples or 1 large
    cooking apple
6 rindless streaky bacon rashers
    (optional)
300ml/½ pint/1¼ cups low-fat
    natural yogurt
15ml/1 tbsp creamed horseradish sauce
sea salt and ground black pepper

1 Preheat the oven to 150°C/300°F/ Gas 2. Mix the onions, fennel, red cabbage and caraway seeds in a bowl. Peel and chop the apples and the bacon rashers, if using, then stir them into the cabbage mixture. Transfer to a casserole. Mix the yogurt with the creamed horseradish sauce.

2 Stir the yogurt and horseradish mixture into the casserole, season with salt and pepper and cover tightly. Bake for 1½ hours, stirring once or twice. Serve hot.

NUTRITION NOTES

Per portion (with bacon):
Energy	158kcals/660kJ
Fat, total	9.7g
saturated fat	3.4g
polyunsaturated fat	1.4g
monounsaturated fat	4.05g
Carbohydrate	12.8g
sugar, total	11.6g
starch	0.2g
Fibre – NSP	4g
Sodium	378mg

Mixed Vegetables with Artichokes

Baking a vegetable medley in the oven is a wonderfully easy way of producing a quick and simple, wholesome mid-week meal.

INGREDIENTS

Serves 4
30ml/2 tbsp olive oil
675g/1½lb frozen broad beans
4 turnips, peeled and sliced
4 leeks, sliced
1 red pepper, seeded and sliced
200g/7oz fresh spinach leaves or
    115g/4oz frozen spinach
2 x 400g/14oz cans artichoke
    hearts, drained
60ml/4 tbsp pumpkin seeds
soy sauce
sea salt and ground black pepper
rice, baked potatoes or wholemeal
    bread, to serve

1 Preheat the oven to 180°C/350°F/ Gas 4. Pour the oil into a casserole. Cook the broad beans in a saucepan of boiling lightly salted water for about 10 minutes. Drain the beans and place them with the turnips, leeks, red pepper slices, spinach and canned artichoke hearts in the casserole.

2 Cover the casserole and bake the vegetables for 30–40 minutes, or until the turnips are soft.

3 Stir in the pumpkin seeds and soy sauce to taste. Season with ground black pepper. Serve solo or with rice sprinkled with chopped fresh herbs, baked potatoes or bread.

NUTRITION NOTES

Per portion:
Energy	335kcals/1410kJ
Fat, total	13.4g
saturated fat	2.2g
polyunsaturated fat	3.3g
monounsaturated fat	6.5g
Carbohydrate	34.95g
sugar, total	11.4g
starch	19.4g
Fibre – NSP	16.3g
Sodium	151.5mg

Wholemeal Pasta with Caraway Cabbage

Crunchy cabbage and Brussels sprouts are the perfect partners for pasta in this healthy dish.

INGREDIENTS

Serves 6
90ml/6 tbsp olive or sunflower oil
3 onions, roughly chopped
350g/12oz round white cabbage, roughly chopped
350g/12oz Brussels sprouts, trimmed and halved
10ml/2 tsp caraway seeds
15ml/1 tbsp chopped fresh dill
400ml/14fl oz/1²/₃ cups vegetable stock
200g/7oz/1³/₄ cups fresh or dried wholewheat pasta spirals
sea salt and ground black pepper
dill sprigs, to garnish

1 Heat the oil in a large saucepan and fry the onions over a low heat for 10 minutes until softened.

2 Add the cabbage and Brussels sprouts and cook for 2–3 minutes, then stir in the caraway seeds and dill. Pour in the stock and season with salt and pepper to taste. Cover and simmer for 5–10 minutes until the cabbage and sprouts are crisp-tender.

— COOK'S TIP —

If tiny baby Brussels sprouts are available they can be used whole for this dish.

3 Meanwhile, cook the pasta in a pan of lightly salted boiling water, following the package instructions, until just tender.

4 Drain the pasta, tip it into a bowl and add the cabbage mixture. Toss lightly, adjust the seasoning and serve.

NUTRITION NOTES	
Per portion:	
Energy	227kcals/953kJ
Fat, total	9.6g
saturated fat	1.4g
polyunsaturated fat	1.5g
monounsaturated fat	5.75g
Carbohydrate	30g
sugar, total	7.65g
starch	21.6g
Fibre – NSP	6.9g
Sodium	53.5mg

Cauliflower and Broccoli with Tomato Sauce

A low-fat alternative to that old favourite, cauliflower cheese. The addition of broccoli to the cauliflower gives extra colour.

INGREDIENTS

Serves 6
1 onion, finely chopped
400g/14oz can chopped tomatoes
45ml/3 tbsp tomato purée
45ml/3 tbsp wholemeal flour
300ml/¹/₂ pint/1¹/₄ cups skimmed milk
300ml/¹/₂ pint/1¹/₄ cups water
1kg/2¹/₄lb/6 cups mixed cauliflower and broccoli florets
sea salt and ground black pepper

1 Mix the onion, tomatoes and tomato purée in a small saucepan. Bring to the boil, lower the heat and simmer for 15–20 minutes.

2 Mix the flour to a paste with a little of the milk. Stir the paste into the tomato mixture, then gradually add the remaining milk and the water. Stir constantly until the mixture boils and thickens. Season to taste with salt and pepper. Keep the sauce hot.

3 Steam the cauliflower (or mixture of cauliflower and broccoli) over boiling water for 5–7 minutes or until the florets are just tender. Tip into a dish, pour over the tomato sauce and serve with extra pepper sprinkled over the top, if liked.

NUTRITION NOTES	
Per portion:	
Energy	116kcals/491kJ
Fat, total	1.85g
saturated fat	0.4g
polyunsaturated fat	0.9g
monounsaturated fat	0.2g
Carbohydrate	16.1g
sugar, total	10.3g
starch	5.4g
Fibre – NSP	4.5g
Sodium	86.8mg

DESSERTS

Desserts are always thought to be a no-go area for diabetics, but modern advice and the judicious use of fruits, mean that diabetics can now eat a wonderful range of desserts. Try, for example, a fruit flan with a tasty yogurt topping, a crumbly oat layer with strawberry filling or a delectable orange cheesecake. The recipes here are sweetened with fruits rather than sugar alternatives, which means that diabetics can absorb the sugar more easily. None-the-less, it is important to remember that most desserts should only be eaten as occasional treats.

Lemon and Walnut Cake

Don't stint on the lemon rind –
it gives this cake a wonderful
zesty tang that complements the
flavour of the walnuts.

INGREDIENTS

Makes a 20cm/8in cake
1 large banana, about 150g/5oz
225g/8oz/1 cup low-fat spread
150g/5oz/scant 1 cup dried,
    stoned dates
5 size 2 eggs
300g/11oz/2³/4 cups wholemeal flour,
    or half wholemeal and half plain
    white flour
75g/3oz/³/4 cup walnut pieces
4 large lemons

1 Preheat the oven to 180°C/350°F/
Gas 4. Lightly grease a deep
20cm/8in loose-based or spring-form
cake tin. Line the base of the tin with
non-stick baking paper.

2 Peel and chop the banana. Process
with the low-fat spread and dates.

3 Add 1 egg and 15ml/1 tbsp of the
flour to the creamed mixture.
Process briefly to mix, then add the
remaining eggs one at a time, each with
a further 15ml/1 tbsp flour.

4 Scrape the mixture into a bowl and
fold in the remaining flour, with
the walnut pieces.

5 Grate the rind from three lemons
and thinly pare the rind from the
fourth (reserve for the decoration).
Squeeze the juice from two lemons,
then stir the grated lemon rind and
juice into the mixture.

6 Spoon the mixture into the
prepared tin. Bake for 50–60
minutes or until a fine skewer inserted
in the centre of the cake comes out
clean. Cool on a wire rack. Decorate
with the pared lemon rind.

───── NUTRITION NOTES ─────

Per cake:	
Energy	2845kcals/11900kJ
Fat, total	163g
saturated fat	34g
polyunsaturated fat	62g
monounsaturated fat	55g
Carbohydrate	280g
sugar, total	90g
starch	190g
Fibre – NSP	34g
Sodium	1660mg

Apple and Cinnamon Cake

Moist and spicy, this is perfect for packed lunches or afternoon tea.

INGREDIENTS

Makes a 20cm/8in square cake

115g/4oz/½ cup low-fat spread, plus extra for greasing
200g/7oz/1¼ cups dried, stoned dates
1–2 tart eating apples or 1 cooking apple, about 225g/8oz
12.5ml/2½ tsp mixed spice
2.5ml/½ tsp salt
75g/3oz/½ cup raisins
2 size 2 eggs, beaten
150g/5oz/1¼ cups wholemeal flour, sifted
115g/4oz/generous 1 cup gram flour, sifted with 10ml/2 tsp baking powder
175ml/6fl oz/¾ cup unsweetened coconut milk

1 Preheat the oven to 180°C/350°F/ Gas 4. Lightly grease a deep 20cm/8in square baking tin and line the base with non-stick baking paper. Combine the low-fat spread and the dates in a food processor. Peel, core and grate the apple or apples and add to the low-fat spread and date mixture with the mixed spice and salt. Process until thoroughly blended.

2 Scrape the apple and date mixture into a bowl and fold in the raisins and beaten eggs alternately with the flours, baking powder and coconut milk. Transfer to the prepared tin and smooth the surface level.

3 Bake for 30–40 minutes until dark golden and firm to the touch. A skewer inserted in the centre should come out clean. Cool the cake in the tin for 15 minutes before turning out on a wire rack to cool completely.

— NUTRITION NOTES —	
Per cake:	
Energy	2036kcals/8588kJ
Fat, total	72g
saturated fat	4.5g
polyunsaturated fat	18.5g
monounsaturated fat	28g
Carbohydrate	300g
sugar, total	150g
starch	147g
Fibre – NSP	34.4g
Sodium	2412mg

Banana Bread

The very ripe bananas that are often sold off cheaply in supermarkets are perfect for this tried and trusted favourite.

INGREDIENTS

Makes 1 loaf
115g/4oz/½ cup low-fat spread, plus
    extra for greasing
5ml/1 tsp bicarbonate of soda
225g/8oz/2 cups wholemeal flour
2 eggs, beaten
3 very ripe bananas
30–45ml/2–3 tbsp unsweetened
    coconut milk or soya milk

1 Preheat the oven to 180°C/350°F/
Gas 4. Grease and base line a
23 x 13cm/9 x 5in loaf tin. Cream the
low-fat spread in a bowl until it is
fluffy. Sift the bicarbonate of soda with
the flour, then add to the creamed low-
fat spread, alternately with the eggs.

NUTRITION NOTES

Per loaf:
Energy	1616kcals/5090kJ
Fat, total	66g
saturated fat	17.5g
polyunsaturated fat	15.2g
monounsaturated fat	26.5g
Carbohydrate	215g
sugar, total	70g
starch	145g
Fibre – NSP	23.5g
Sodium	2320mg

2 Peel the bananas and slice them
into a bowl. Mash them well, then
stir them into the cake mixture. Mix in
the coconut milk or soya milk.

VARIATION

Sunflower seeds make a good addition to
banana cake. Add about 50g/2oz/½ cup to
the mixture just before baking.

3 Spoon the mixture into the loaf tin
and level the surface with a spoon.
Bake for about 1¼ hours or until a fine
skewer inserted in the centre comes out
clean. Cool on a wire rack.

Flapjacks

Perfect for picnics and packed lunches, these flapjacks are really crisp and crunchy.

INGREDIENTS

Makes 16
115g/4oz/½ cup low-fat spread
60ml/4 tbsp rice syrup
50g/2oz/½ cup wholemeal flour
225g/8oz/2 cups porridge oats
50g/2oz/⅔ cup pine nuts

1 Preheat the oven to 180°C/350°F/ Gas 4. Line a 20cm/8in shallow baking tin with oiled foil. Melt the low-fat spread and rice syrup in a small saucepan over a low heat, then stir in the flour, porridge oats and pine nuts until well mixed.

2 Tip the mixture into the tin and pat it out evenly with your fingers. Press the mixture down lightly. Bake for 25–30 minutes until the flapjacks are lightly browned and crisp. Mark into squares while still warm. Cool slightly, then lift them out of the tin and cool on a wire rack.

— COOK'S TIP —

Do not let the syrup mixture boil or the flapjacks will be tacky rather than crisp.

— NUTRITION NOTES —

Per flapjack:
Energy	122kcals/513kJ
Fat, total	6.4g
saturated fat	1.2g
polyunsaturated fat	2.55g
monounsaturated fat	2.35g
Carbohydrate	14.3g
sugar, total	1.45g
starch	11.05g
Fibre – NSP	1.35g
Sodium	54.1mg

Ginger Biscuits

INGREDIENTS

Makes 8 gingerbread men or 10–12 biscuits
115g/4oz/1 cup plain flour, sifted
7.5ml/1½ tsp ground ginger
grated rind of 1 orange and 1 lemon
75ml/5 tbsp pear and apple spread
25g/1oz/2 tbsp low-fat spread
16 currants and 8 raisins, to
    decorate (optional)

— NUTRITION NOTES —

Per gingerbread man:
Energy	85kcals/360kJ
Fat, total	1.5g
saturated fat	0.4g
polyunsaturated fat	0.5g
monounsaturated fat	0.55g
Carbohydrate	17.25g
sugar, total	5.85g
starch	11.4g
Fibre – NSP	0.5g
Sodium	23.1mg

1 Preheat the oven to 180°C/350°F/ Gas 4. Mix the sifted flour, ginger and grated orange and lemon rind in a bowl. Melt the pear and apple spread and the low-fat spread in a small saucepan over a low heat.

2 As soon as the pear and apple spread and margarine mixture has melted, stir it into the dry ingredients. Mix to a firm dough in the bowl, then remove the dough, wrap it in clear film and chill for 2–3 hours.

3 Roll out the dough on a lightly floured surface to a thickness of about 5mm/¼in. Cut out gingerbread men, using a cutter or a template. Alternatively, stamp the dough into 10–12 rounds with a 7cm/2¾in cutter.

4 If making gingerbread men, give them currant eyes and raisin noses. Using the point of a knife, draw a mouth on each. Place the biscuits on a lightly floured baking sheet and bake for 8–10 minutes. Cool on a wire rack.

Fruit and Nut Chocolates

When beautifully boxed, these make perfect presents.

INGREDIENTS

Makes 20

50g/2oz ready-to-eat stoned prunes or dried apricots
50g/2oz/⅓ cup sultanas or raisins
25g/1oz/2 tbsp ready-to eat dried apples, figs or dates
25g/1oz/⅓ cup flaked almonds
25g/1oz/¼ cup hazelnuts or walnuts
30–60ml/2–4 tbsp lemon juice
50g/2oz good-quality dark chocolate

1 Chop the fruit and nuts in a food processor or blender until fairly small. Add 30ml/2 tbsp lemon juice and process again to mix. Scrape the mixture into a bowl, taste and add more lemon juice if needed.

2 Melt the chocolate in a heatproof bowl over simmering water. Roll the fruit mixture into small balls. Using tongs or two forks, roll the balls in the melted chocolate, then place them on oiled foil to cool and set. If the chocolate becomes too solid to work with, reheat it gently.

NUTRITION NOTES

Per chocolate:

Energy	42kcals/176kJ
Fat, total	2.3g
saturated fat	0.55g
polyunsaturated fat	0.8g
monounsaturated fat	0.8g
Carbohydrate	4.95g
sugar, total	4.85g
starch	0.05g
Fibre – NSP	0.5g
Sodium	1.9mg

Apple and Date Balls

INGREDIENTS

Makes 20

1kg/2¼lb cooking apples or pears
115g/4oz/⅔ cup dried, stoned dates
250ml/8fl oz/1 cup apple juice
5ml/1 tsp ground cinnamon
50g/2oz/½ cup finely chopped walnuts

NUTRITION NOTES

Per ball:

Energy	47kcals/198kJ
Fat, total	1.8g
saturated fat	0.15g
polyunsaturated fat	1.25g
monounsaturated fat	0.3g
Carbohydrate	7.6g
sugar, total	7.6g
starch	0g
Fibre – NSP	1g
Sodium	1.9mg

1 Halve the unpeeled fruit and place in a large heavy-based saucepan. Add the dates, apple juice and ground cinnamon. Cook over a very low heat, stirring occasionally, for 4–6 hours or until the mixture forms a dry paste. Scrape into a bowl and cool, then roll the mixture into bite-sized balls. Toast the nuts under the grill until golden.

2 Coat the balls in the nut mixture. Twist each ball in a sweet wrapper or cellophane; store in an airtight box.

VARIATION

Use half-and-half ground cinnamon and ginger instead of the 5ml/1 tsp cinnamon.

Wholemeal Cheese Scones

These are very good warm with a little sunflower margarine.

INGREDIENTS

Makes 15
450g/1lb/4 cups wholemeal flour
pinch of salt
10ml/2 tsp baking powder
115g/4oz Parmesan cheese,
 finely grated
50g/2oz/¼ cup sunflower margarine
150–300ml/¼–½ pint/²⁄₃–1¼ cups
 buttermilk (see Cook's Tip)

—————— COOK'S TIP ——————

If you cannot obtain buttermilk, sour skimmed milk by stirring in a generous squeeze of lemon juice. Let the mixture stand for about 10 minutes before using it.

1 Preheat the oven to 200°C/400°F/ Gas 6. Mix the flour, salt, baking powder and Parmesan cheese in a bowl and rub in the margarine with your fingertips until the mixture resembles breadcrumbs. Working quickly and lightly, stir in enough of the buttermilk to make a moist dough.

2 Pat out the dough on a lightly floured board to a thickness of about 4cm/1½ in.

3 Using a 7cm/2¾ in cutter, cut out 15 rounds. Place the rounds on a floured baking sheet and bake for about 10 minutes. The exact cooking time will depend on the depth of the scones. They should be well risen and lightly browned. Serve warm, cut in half, with a little sunflower margarine.

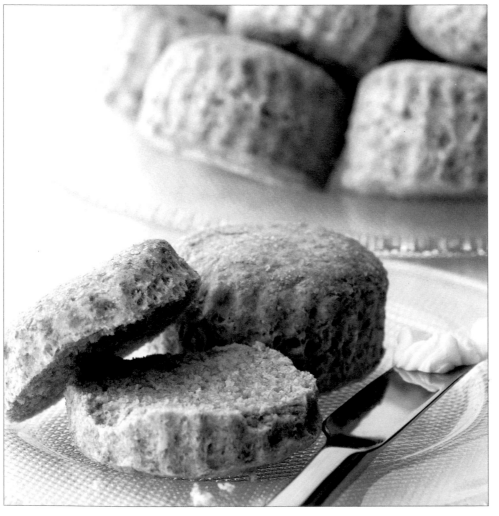

—————— NUTRITION NOTES ——————

Per scone:
Energy	160kcals/674kJ
Fat, total	5.95g
saturated fat	2.25g
polyunsaturated fat	1.55g
monounsaturated fat	1.7g
Carbohydrate	20.4g
sugar, total	1.65g
starch	18.8g
Fibre – NSP	2.7g
Sodium	196.6mg

Information File

FURTHER READING

Beat Sugar Craving
by Maryon Stewart – Vermilion
Diabetes – A New Guide
by Dr Rowan Hillson – Optima
Healing Foods
by Miriam Polunin – Dorling
    Kindersley
Nutritional Medicine
by Dr Stephen Davies and Dr Alan
    Stewart – Pan Books
The Diabetic Kids' Cookbook
by Jane Rossiter and Rosemary
Seddon – Optima
The Inside Story on Food & Health
Subscription magazine with general
information on diet and nutrition and
a lot of original, tested, no added
sugar, low-fat, dairy-free recipes.
Available from:
Berrydales Publishers
5 Lawn Road
London NW3 2 XS
Tel: 0171 722 2866

HELPFUL ORGANIZATIONS

The main associations dealing with
diabetes. Helplines, magazines, research
material, etc.

British Diabetic Association
10 Queen Anne's Street
London W1M OBD
Tel: 0171 323 1531
Canadian Diabetic Association
15 Toronto Street
Suite 800
Toronto
Ontario M5C2E3
Tel: Freephone 1 (800) Banting
Diabetes Australia
National Office
5–7 Phipps Place
Deakin ACT 2615
Tel: Freephone 1 (800) 640 862
South African Diabetes Association
PO Box 1715
Saxonwold 21342
Tel: 011 (788) 45 95

Institute For Complementary Medicine,
PO Box 194,
London SE16 1QZ
Tel: 0171 237 5165
Register of qualified complementary
practitioners. Public referral service,
newsletter and research material.
Medic Alert Foundation,
1 Bridge Wharf,
156 Caledonian Road,
London N1 9UU
Tel: 0171 833 3034
Emergency identification system for
people with diabetes, allergies or other
hidden medical problems.

SHORT GLOSSARY OF BASIC TERMS

Adrenalin – hormone produced by
the adrenal gland to combat physical or
nervous stress.
Arteriosclerosis – hardening up or
furring up of the arteries.
Blood glucose – glucose level in
the blood (also known as blood
sugar), usually elevated in the case
of diabetics.
Cystitis – inflammation of the bladder.
Diabetes Mellitus – condition where
the blood sugar level is above normal.
Diuretics – pills that increase
urination.
Glucose – simple sugar found in
carbohydrates providing one of the
main energy sources for the body.
Glycogen – the form in which
glucose is stored in the blood.
Glycosuria – sugar or glucose in the
urine.
Hyperglycaemia – too much sugar or
glucose in the blood.
Hypoglycaemia – too little sugar or
glucose in the blood.
Insulin – hormone produced in the
pancreas, which allows glucose to enter
the blood stream.
Insulin Dependent Diabetes – a
condition in which the pancreas stops
producing insulin. The only treatment
is injected insulin.
Insulin receptor – site on the surface
of a cell into which the insulin

"docks" in order to allow the glucose
to enter through the cell walls.
Juvenile onset diabetes – diabetes
starting in youth that is nearly always
insulin dependent.
Ketoacidosis – severe excess of
glucose in the blood due to a severe
insulin deficiency causing fat breakdown and ketone formation.
Ketones – products that result from fat
breakdown that, in turn, results from
severe insulin deficiency. They smell of
acetone and are a symptom of severe
hyperglycaemia.
Maturity onset diabetes – diabetes
that affects people over 30 and that is
not usually insulin dependent.
Neuropathy – an abnormality in the
functioning of the nerves. Autonomic
neuropathy is partial failure of the
nerves controlling automatic body
functions. Peripheral Neuropathy
means that the nerves in the arms and
legs are affected.
Non Insulin Dependent Diabetes –
a condition where the pancreas is still
producing insulin, but either it is not
producing enough or is not acting very
effectively. Can usually be treated with
diet and glucose-lowering drugs.
Pancreas – a gland that is found
behind the stomach but in front of the
backbone. The pancreas produces
insulin and other digestive hormones.
Polydipsia – drinking large amounts
of water.
Polyuria – passing excessive amounts
of water on a frequent basis.
Retinopathy – abnormality of retina
in the eye, often caused by diabetes.

Index